LIVING WITH SICKLE CELL CHILDREN:

THE VOICE

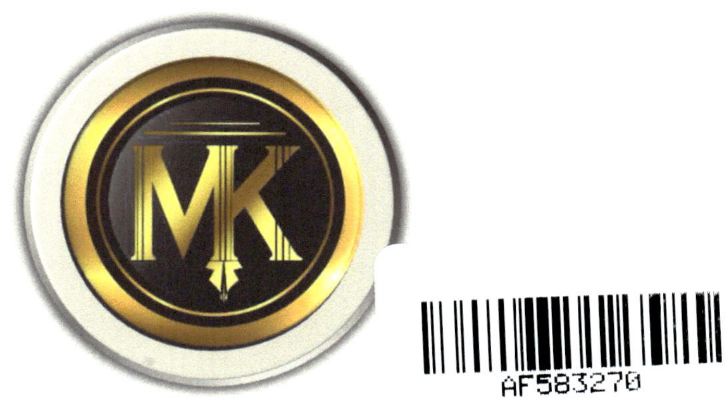

MEMORY MWANZA

&

KENNEDY MWANZA

AUTHOR

FOREWORD

My Name is Memory Mwanza and I was born on 27th December 1983 in Zambia Africa. I spent most of my life in Zambia. Having completed my course in 2006, I found a job in one of the Banks in Zambia which I enjoyed.

In 2006 my then boyfriend now husband Kennedy Mwanza decided to come to the UK to study and in 2007 he organized for me to come and study for my degree course here in the UK. On arrival, I reported to the school and found a job with an agency and I was sent to work in a warehouse, I must say I did some of the easy jobs there and it was fun as I got to work in different warehouses. Life was not easy as I had to study and work.

I moved on to work for the UK government after completing my studies and I am now working for one of the Banks.

My husband and I got married in 2008 and we have four lovely boys, they all came as a blessing to us as you will see while reading this book. They have been our tower as we wouldn't be where we are without them. We always give thanks to our God for this blessing.

We have decided to write a book about sickle cell because of the struggles we have experienced and what we found helpful. Our hope is one day the book will reach someone going through the same and find the comfort that it will work out for them as it was for us with the help of God our creator. Also, we might help someone with the proceeds from the book.

Dedication

I would like to dedicate this book to my one and forever husband Kennedy Mwanza the father of our four boys, who has been a pillar at all times, and without him, this book would not have been written. He has written most of the stories in this book. Our first son Aaron Mwansa Mwanza, without him there would be no story to tell. He has suffered and has come out stronger and it pleasures our hearts because he knows God Jehovah did it for him. We call him our saviour because we wouldn't be where we are now without him. Our second son Carwyn Mwenya Mwanza, is such a person you would want to spend the whole time with. The little discussions he comes up with, we would have forgotten some of the stories in the book without him. Our third son Eirian Mayamiko Mwanza's arrival made our life a little bit more different. He is such a beautiful person with a soft heart, a person who knows what he wants even at his age (2years). He can pray to God and no one can take it away. It is such a joy. Our last born Gavi Chimwemwe Mwanza, just by the meaning of his name which you will find in the book. He has brought joy to our hearts and he is the one to bring us a lot closer to God. At 15 months he can praise God and can say Hallelujah.

We want to say a big thank you to the Nurses and doctors at Northampton General hospital including consultant's Dr. Ali, Dr. Koodiyedath and Dr. Breene, Specialist nurse Claire Stockley. Leicester Royal infirmary Hospital all the nurses and doctors that were involved in the care of our son Aaron Mwansa Mwanza and Birmingham children's hospital, Nurses and doctors from nearly every department of the hospital including his consultant Dr. Lawson and his ex-consultant Dr. Derbyshire. With their support and efforts with our sons, we are so grateful to them and only God will reward them in his own way.

My mother Maud Mwenya without her I wouldn't be who I am. I have learned a lot from her, one of the things is to be strong and put God at the heart of everything. My siblings including my late big sister Audrey (RIP) made their efforts to call and encourage us throughout my struggles.

My mother-in-law for the support and all of my husband's family that were there for us. Auntie Bridget thank you as without her we would not have known about the treatment.

A thank also to my friend Petronella who was there at the time of need. She helped with child care when Mwansa was in Birmingham Hospital and also for the visits that she gave us while in Northampton hospital. Thank you Prosperlyn and Chitalu who we now call mother and sister for the support.

Everyone needs a spiritual person in their lives, Pastor Shadrack and his Wife Pastor Natalia have been a big help in our lives. The prayers they render on our behalf. Thank you, Pastors may God bless their ministry.

Edgar Mtonga and his wife Cornelia for their support both emotionally and finally. The prosperous ladies who supported us emotionally and financially. Lauren Pell for her support. Patricial Bimbe thank you for all the support you have rendered to our family. My boys think you are my blood sister. Anniestazia and the boys Ntemesha Kachiza and Wana Kachiza thank you for all the support.

We would like to thank Ronald McDonalds house in Birmingham for its support. They accommodated us throughout the time we got admitted to the hospital.

Table of Contents

CHAPTER 1

I am the 6th born in a family of 7. Growing up I never saw anyone in my family with sickle cell and I had no idea that I was a carrier. On the other hand, my husband had no one in the family that suffered from sickle cell. People with sickle cell disease produce unusually shaped blood cells that can cause problems because they do not live as long as healthy blood cells and can block blood vessels.

Like everyone normally says, things happen for a reason. I met Kennedy my now husband in Zambia and he travelled to UK and I followed a year after.

We got married and looked forward to having kids. We got pregnant and unfortunately, just after 8 weeks, we lost the baby. Got pregnant again and the same thing happened at 8 weeks. Again, we got pregnant this time even more worried and at 8 weeks we lost the baby. They checked our bloods to see why this kept on happening at the same stage of pregnancy and also whether we were compatible. Unfortunately, the bloods did not show anything.

The Heartbeat

Months went by and this time we thought of giving up then, we got pregnant and we were more worried than ever before. At 6 weeks I felt stomach pains. I told my husband that I needed to see the doctor as I didn't feel well and we thought the worst again, while at the hospital they decided to do a scan. And there is the heartbeat, showed us the baby and we were happy for the first time to see a heartbeat there but we were worried. Eight weeks came and gone we kept hoping for the best.

It was routine blood test time and I went to the midwife's appointment. She took the blood samples and after a few days she called me back to come and see her with my husband. We got to the surgery and she told us that all the other blood results were fine apart from one which was sickle cell. She explained what it was and advised that they needed to test my husband to check whether he also had the trait or he had full sickle cell (SS). She took the bloods on the same day.

A few days later the midwife called to say we needed to go and see her, she confirmed he was also a carrier. At the time we were not so bothered as she said that there was a 1 in 4 chance the baby would be a sickle cell carrier or full (SS). She advised that they test people in pregnancy to see whether the baby would be carrying sickle cell and she explained the procedure. They would put a needle through the belly to get to the baby and she said there could be some complications which includes miscarriage.

I will not allow the injection through me and to our baby to take the blood samples. What if it comes out positive and I don't want to terminate? Meaning I would be thinking and stressing throughout the pregnancy. And miscarriage was not a word we ever wanted to hear because of what we went through. Whatever comes, it's a gift from God we said. We had mixed feelings and emotions but we trusted God, our baby would be fine. And luckily my husband felt the same about the test. The nurse advised we don't have to do anything if we so wished, it's just something they offered. We decided not to do the test.

Baby Arrived

Three months later at 32 weeks, I had an appointment with the midwife and after cleaning the house I went to see her. Memory do you have anyone that can take you to the hospital? Now what? My heart started racing. What's wrong I asked, your BP is very high and we can't let you go on your own the midwife advised. So, you will need to sit down and call for someone she said. Kennedy was working and luckily my friend Charity was off that day. I called her and she came to the surgery and took me to the hospital. I was so grateful for her as she was also pregnant but she gave up her resting time to take me to the hospital.

As I was over 30 weeks, I was required to go straight to the labour ward. Memory, you have pre-eclampsia and we will need to keep an eye on you. I stayed in the labour ward the whole day. We will give you steroids just to help with the baby's lungs. I had no idea they were preparing me for delivery. In the evening the nurse told me that they were going to transfer me to the maternity ward. They kept me and I was on monitors and the baby. The doctors kept coming to check on me. One of the doctors who dealt with Jehovah's witnesses (I was going to JW at the time and signed no blood forms) was one of the doctors that came to see me. On the third day he came and said we have done what we can to stabilize your BP but it is not going down and due to your faith, we need to do something quickly before we are left with no options. There was a bit of conflict of information, one doctor said to my husband and me that we do not need to rush in the decision as it has not reached a scare point and another was worried because of the blood. On the fourth day, the decision was made to deliver the baby through C-Section. For some reason I did not respond to the first anaesthetic, the doctor was like Memory lift your leg and I did straight away, they waited for a little bit and asked again and I raised the leg. My husband was with me holding my hand. We looked at each other and even though he smiled I could see the worry in his eyes. They decided to give me another dose and it worked. And at 32/4 days they delivered baby Aaron weighing 1.5 kg through C section around 11 am memories still fresh. Memory, meet your son and in no time baby Aaron was taken away in an incubator to the neonatal unit and I was taken to another ward.

Gosset Baby unit

Because of the amount of anaesthetics they gave me, I slept the whole day and could not move my legs. My husband went to see the baby and took pictures. The following morning, I recovered from anaesthetics. I told the nurse on the ward that I wanted to see the baby. The nurse called for the hospital porter and he took me in the wheelchair, my husband was with me. We got to the ward which was full of incubators with tiny babies. As we walked, I kept on looking for my baby till we reached him and saw the real tiny baby connected to wires in an incubator. I looked at my husband and just broke down. Not knowing Kennedy was also asking himself whether Mwansa will make it? He says because there were many, he quickly answered himself that he will. A lot of things started going around in my head, I was asking myself whether my baby would make it? I thank God because Kennedy was there with me.

There was a belief in me that he will make it, but I was so worried. I was not sure to touch him but he was my baby and I wanted him to know I was there. The nurse looked at me and said, it is ok to touch him and he will know his mummy is there. I put my hand through the tiny window and held him and said hello to him.

The nurse explained that the baby settled well but he had jaundice which was why he had the lights on him, with the face covered to protect his eyes. He was initially on c pup (breathing support machine) when he was born because the doctors thought he would need it as he was too small at only 1.5kg but they took it off just after a few hours of being in the baby unit. The nurse said he was a strong boy even though you see him as this small. This somehow comforted us. I looked around and there were about 3/4 other babies in the same room some with the lights on like Aaron.

The nurse asked us how we were going to feed the baby, was it going to be breastfeeding or bottle feeding? I told the nurse I will breastfeed. I looked at the tiny baby and thought would he be able to drink? They advised pumping some milk and store in the fridge for the nurses to use when we were not there. I would lift and feed him but most of the time it was through the tube this was to make sure he was feeding enough.

The doctors would come round to check on the baby and feedback on how he was doing. Then, the doctors called and advised that the baby will potentially remain in the hospital even when I was discharged until he reached his full term and he was able to maintain body weight, temperature, and feed well. Meaning over 2 months. Imagine that mothers and fathers. They reassured us they would do their best to make sure he was comfortable and was growing well also that we could call and visit him at any time. This meant living him all by himself and also for us commuting. I got discharged and we visited the baby every day. Our house was not far from the hospital and we usually walked but it was hard especially for me with the scar from the C section. Unfortunately, just after few days after getting discharged the scar started to open on the side and this was painful.

What helped us through all this was our prayers and the faith we had that God will see us through also the love we have for each other also our love for our baby.

Diagnosis

They took blood samples from the baby to check for sickle cell among other things. We dreaded the results and we tried not to be affected by them but it was hard. While in the hospital we spoke to one of the Chinese dads who had a baby there and he said his son had been there for over 4 months. We felt sorry and did not know what to say. But they helped us emotionally, as they showed us the size of how their baby was and how big he became. Kennedy looked at nurses happily looking after all those helpless babies and just said well.

We were allowed to have close family to visit. At the time my brother-in-law Kenny and his wife Mei were around (they have now migrated to Japan) and they gave us support. But as we are far away from our families who are in Zambia, we consider friends as family as they fill that missing part. One of our friends visited and we explained the situation and that we were waiting for the blood results. We are not sure up to today whether it was intentional or not, but they started talking about one of the husband's relatives that suffered from sickle cell. We felt upset about it but never said anything as we were not sure what to say to them, to not make them feel uncomfortable. We just said why would they be telling someone in our situation the negative things and this went on for a while. They would both be telling how that person got sick all the time and was always in hospital. Kennedy told me to stop them and even when the results came, we never told them until after a while. We felt they were not good and supportive friends.

Five days later they told us our worst fears, it was confirmed he was sickle cell positive. It was a Sad Day even though we didn't understand the impact at the time but the Doctor said normally he will not show any signs of sickle cell until after 6 months, when the blood he was born with and the ant bodies from the mother finished. And also, that sickle cell affects people differently. Some may suffer from anaemia, joint pain, stomach pain, chest and other things. Other may live with it without any symptoms. And we hoped for the best with Mwansa.

Mwansa stayed in hospital for 3 weeks and he was discharged because he was doing so well that the doctors were surprised. We took our Mwansa home in a car seat and you could barely see him in it as he was very small. We welcomed him home and our journey with him began. He got in a routine and our baby was growing just like other babies except he was tiny. He would sleep and woke up for feeds. We were happy at last.

CHAPTER 2

The Struggle started

You may see the first signs at 6 months the doctors advised and we did not think it would be that. We noticed his eyes looked yellow but we did not know how serious it was as this was all new to us, if we did, we would have taken him to the hospital. We did not think it was something we were to be worried for. On the 8/10/2011, I stayed with Mwansa as hubby was working like I always did and I was playing with him. I even put him on the over door swing and he was giggling. Night time came and I put him to bed. I normally cleaned in the night to have my time with him during the day and I did the same on the night. He would normally wake up at midnight to feed and this is what he did on that night I thought. I looked at the time it was not quite midnight it was about 9pm.

I just finished cleaning (I was dry cleaning the carpet) and he woke up crying. I went to feed him, he fed a little but then carried on crying, I turned to Kennedy who usually woke up with me to feed our baby and I told him something was not right and rang the out of hours doctors but as usual the receptionist told us the doctors would call back but they took so long to call. His breathing changed and we decided to go to the hospital, we were not driving at the time so we called a taxi.

We were just locking the door when the doctor rang, by this time his breathing had changed, I made him listen to his breathing but he just said since you have already booked for a taxi you can come but ambulance would have been called (he should have said, stay at home and wait for the ambulance as he was experienced to know the breathing was not right) we were just new parents and had never called ambulance for anything and we didn't understand what was happening with our baby. The doctor could have picked up on the breathing and advised correctly.

We got to the out of hours and we were told to wait. When we got there one of the doctors was at the reception desk and he must have heard how our baby was breathing but he finished what he was there for and left. The feet started getting cold I went to the receptionist and she said just wait. I got back where Kennedy was sitting and I started crying. Kennedy got Mwansa and walked towards the reception and I walked to follow him and he looked at me quizzical. Few minutes later Mwansa stopped breathing and eyes rolled back. Kennedy said Memory I think, look and I put my fingers on his nose to check whether he was breathing and I just started shouting for help and pushed the doors to the doctor's rooms. One of the doctors came out and rushed Mwansa in one of the rooms, cut his clothes and started CPR using 2 fingers as he was just a small baby.

We were in such a shock; Kennedy was crying and I was just busy talking to God. I was telling him not to allow the devil to take our child. He gave us the baby after such a struggle and this was not something, we were ready to accept. The doctor called for help and they called an Ambulance. The Ambulance came just after few minutes and they took over CPR and they also used a Defibrillator and Mwansa started breathing but very faintly. They took Mwansa in the big Ambulance to the hospital accident and emergency which was just on the other side of the road and we were driven in a small response ambulance in the early hours of 9/11/2011.

We got to the hospital and we were taken to resuscitation room where Mwansa was and they were trying to find a way to transfuse fluids and blood. His blood was just 1.5 litres when it should have been 10 litres. All his veins had collapsed and they tried every way, they even cut his hair on the sides and still there was no veins. We could see the frustration in the doctors as they wanted this boy to live. We were still praying for our baby. It looked like they had done all they could and was about to stop, then one doctor stood up and said there's one more thing we could do, we could drill his bones without anaesthetic and give blood through there. He quickly run to find the drill and they called me closer to hold his hand.

They drilled the bone in the legs and our boy who was so week held me so tightly to tell me it was painful and that was not easy to see. I tried to comfort him and just felt the need to take his pain for him but of course it was not possible. Kennedy was behind me trying to calm me down. My husband broke down.

They managed to put the canula and transfused water straight away and they were preparing for blood. The doctors kept coming to us to tell us what they were doing. And one of the doctors came to say they will need to put bloods and they also needed blood from me as he might need some antibodies. But then he remembered the notes said I was going to Jehovah's witness and I had said no to transfusion for me. But Kennedy was a Catholic and he was fine with blood transfusion also as Mwansa was a baby the hospital (government) had the right to decide for him. I initially said no then I changed my mind and said I will give him. They said they were not going to let me go against my wish and reassured us that even if they don't get my bloods, they were going to use other medications that would help him. And they started the transfusion of both water and blood.

God and Faith

What helped us through all this was our prayers and the faith we had that God will see us through, also the love we have for each other.

While all this was going on, other doctors were making arrangements for Mwansa to be taken to another hospital in Leicester royal infirmary hospital. Other doctors were working on stabilising Mwansa. Others were making sure we were well informed of every step. After connecting the fluids, the doctor came and took us to one of the parent's rooms to show us were to get a drink and to talk to us about what had happened and what plan they had.

They advised that they were going to send Mwansa to Leicester because Northampton General Hospital have no ventilators and other machines that monitors children.

Leicester Royal Infirmary was one of the specialist hospitals that looks after children that needs intensive care.

We finished the conversation with the doctor and went back to the resuscitation room where Mwansa was. We didn't think about drinks at all. Minutes later, this was about 5am the nurse and one of the senior Paediatric consultants from Leicester arrived. They introduced us and the hand over started. They took Mwansa in a special Ambulance I never saw before they called it critical care Ambulance and we were not allowed in that ambulance. They gave us the address and advised we could go there straight away. It was hard to see him taken away without us, our baby Mwansa was all by himself.

The walk home was another thing, we had never felt so helpless. We pushed an empty pushchair. We stood at the door, looked at each other and that was just another feeling we never felt before. It was painful! We went in the house and there was silence. Baby Mwansa's voice was not there. We had the fear not knowing he would come back but we had a belief he will be ok. This was the hardest thing we experienced.

We got ready packed the little things we needed and we went to Leicester Royal Infirmary hospital. We got to the hospital and the nurse took us to see Aaron. We walked to his room and we were greeted with a baby wrapped up in cables of medication that were running through his tiny veins and had a tube to help him breath. His face swollen because of the number of fluids that he had and he was immobile. Of course, I broke down because that was not the best to see of your own child. The nurse explained to us what they were doing with him and they were very helpful. They told us they are doing all they can to get him better and all we could do is have faith he would be fine. The nurse left us in the room and we prayed with Mwansa. We believed God will make him better.

The nurse came back to show us our room and told us we could visit the baby anytime even in the night. We prayed in the room they gave us which was just outside intensive care unit. And I could get up in the night to check on baby Mwansa. My baby needed milk but he could not feed because he had the tube in the mouth, I would express and give to the nurse to keep in the fridge. The trust in God kept us going.

Recovery

Three days later, he was moved to the main intensive care ward where he stayed for about 10 days. Praise God our baby was going to be ok. We did not think he would make it and we were just trying our best the nurse said. He is a strong boy and you are lucky parents. The doctors would come to speak to us to tell us what they were doing and his progress. They told us that because he had a period of oxygen starvation to his brain for few minutes when he stopped breathing, he might have brain damage and might not be able to walk, talk and might be bed ridden. They were going to do MRI scan to his brain to check how his brain was doing.

The doctors were saying all this in my heart I was just saying he will be fine, God kept him and he will heal him. My God is faithful and he keeps to His promise. He gave us Mwansa and He did give us.

Then slowly he started moving limbs and one day he opened his eyes and we thanked God. MRI scan was done and the good news was his brain was not damaged as they initially expected due to lack of oxygen. The Doctor said it was remarkable you guys and the baby are lucky. Yes, because God was there through out. They explained to us that the Spleen sucked up the blood and that was what made him so unwell (A spleen is an organ in the body that help fight infections, with sickle cell the spleen thinks it's the infection and this is what led to it trapping the blood).

Discharged

Mwansa was going in the right recovery direction. We were moved out of intensive care to a normal ward and we were expected to stay a little longer in that ward but because of the progress he was making just on the second day in the ward the doctor came and said they were discharging Mwansa, they gave us an option to either go home or go to Northampton General Hospital. We chose home because the doctors said they were not worried of anything and even if we went to Northampton hospital, they would not keep him. They were going to arrange transport back to Northampton and they would discuss with Northampton Hospital of Mwansa's progress. And just about 15 days in hospital Mwansa was home. We got home and it felt right our baby was home.

We then had a review with Dr Ali and he told us that we had an open access to Disney ward at Northampton General Hospital (Anyone with certain complications had open access). We were not to take Mwansa to A & E but straight to Disney as most Paediatricians would be there. We wished we were told from day one and maybe Mwansa would not have gone through what he went through. But again, everything happens for a reason.

CHAPTER 3

The battle with sickle cell did not end there. The journey had just began. Our life was always on the edge. We were constantly checking whether our boy was ok. Mwansa was sick a lot. Northampton general hospital and Birmingham children's hospital was our second home. He spent most of the time between Northampton and Birmingham children hospital. Some time we would go to Northampton General Hospital and Kennedy would go back alone pushing an empty push chair because Mwansa and I would be taken to Birmingham children hospital by ambulance. Very sad it used to be.

The difficult to find his veins to take or transfuse fluids (water, blood and medication) was distressing and painful to see. Because junior Doctors would attempt 2 times and still not manage and I would come out of the treatment room crying leaving Kennedy to comfort Mwansa. It normally took consultants to deal with it (cannula).

The mile stones were also affected, being born prematurely and the amount of time he spent in the hospital. The moment he started getting confident to craw he would be hit by a crisis which would keep him bedridden for some days. Our boy was slow in everything (development). We understood his situation and we did not stress about it. We just knew he would get there. We trusted God would do it for him. Mwansa was small and some children that were born around his time looked so much bigger than him, they did most of the milestones that he did not. Some people made fun of that but we didn't allow it to get to us.

Sometimes people would look amazed by how small he was and they would stair but again we didn't allow it to get to us. Some people did not know how our life was like and they didn't understand how much Mwansa had achieved. We were always proud of our boy. He always tried his best to get to his mile stone, he sometimes had fear of failing when he tried to stand and walk. Every time he started doing one thing, he would fall sick and would stay in the hospital for a week, taking him back to square one. We would help him build the confidence. We lived in a block of flats and we had a clean corridor where we would take him to learn to walk. And one day he just walked. That was the best feeling we felt. Our God is good.

Blood Transfusions

Mwansa was put on 4 weeks blood transfusion and as we said finding his veins was crucial, the Doctor suggested for a pot. This is the tube which is connected to the main vain and the pot inserted underneath the skin below the chest. It makes it easy to get and transfuse fluids by nurses instead of waiting for doctors. Our boy has had approximately over 70 times of blood not from me or my husband but from unrelated donor. Therefore, I encourage everyone to consider being a blood donor not only for sickle cell patients but for every one especially black and other ethnic minority. His bloods came from all over the country.

I did not believe in blood transfusion because of the scripture in the bible (Acts) that says do not eat blood (my understanding was that if a patient can't feed from the mouth and is fed through the tube, we normally say he's fed through the tube, so blood transfusion is feeding through the tube. I had a change of mind because if people get cured because of having a transfusion the blood should be considered as medication. This issue is confusing for me up to now but I believe one day God will make things clear to me.

Any way we read about the pot and spoke to some family who had a similar situation. We accepted to have it done on Mwansa. On 18th August 2012 we went to have it put on at Birmingham children hospital and this made transfusion better.

CHAPTER 4

Splenectomy

Everything seemed to be going on well for some time. Then, the issue of Spleen which nearly killed him for good became a major issue. We mentioned about the Spleen earlier but We did not explain what it was in detail. So, the spleen plays multiple supporting roles in the body. It acts as a filter for blood as part of the immune system. Old red blood cells are recycled in the spleen, and platelets and white blood cells are stored there. The spleen also helps fight certain kinds of bacteria that cause pneumonia and meningitis. Because of sickle cell the spleen tends to trap the blood cell causing someone to be anaemic. This was usually the case with Mwansa and he used to get chest infections quite a lot.

The doctors decided that he should have it removed and August 2012 we went to Birmingham Children's hospital and Mwansa had his second operation. The Spleen was removed. This did not solve the problem completely. Mwansa still got chest infections with wizziness that required Nebulizers. We would go for a quick check up in our minds but will come back home after nearly a week in hospital because he needed Nebulizer and oxygen. Life was not easy.

Kennedy thought I managed the situation well, as he struggled and did not want to talk about it not even to the family. Every time he went out and specially to have his hair cut, people would be asking why our son's eyes were yellow or looked tired. In the end he started cutting Mwansa's hair at home. With time he managed to speak to some few family members. Thankfully, Auntie Bridget told him about one story of her friend's child that got cured in America. Then, we had a review with Dr Ali and Dr Derbyshire, we asked them and they said they will put him on the donor register. They warned, it's not always easy to find a donor especially for people from ethnic minority. They went on to say the procedure is complex and there are risks which includes death.

Breaking Point

Kennedy did not realise I was at breaking point. I looked at my son I did not know what I could do to take the pain away from him. I blamed myself for bringing him in this world. It felt like I brought him to come and suffer. On the other hand, I looked at Kennedy and I thought both of us cannot be weak one has to be strong to see us through. I would go out of both their sights to cry and come back like nothing happened. I would cry when having my shower, I would cry in the kitchen. I had so many secret tears that Kennedy didn't see. I did not want our son to feel the stress in both of us. I wanted him strong and I spoke to him about God. As I couldn't pull myself without God. So much had happened and I still trusted and still trust God has a very big reason for all this. My mind was constantly thinking why me? Of all my siblings but me? God surely has a reason.

Dilated Heart

As if sickle cell was not enough, the doctors told us Mwansa had a dilated heart and this could be because of sickle cell. We were always on tip toes not knowing what next. They put him on close monitor and they scan his heart every year.

The doctors put Mwansa on X-jade, one of the medications they use in cancer treatment. I did not fully understand the medication, all I knew was it was to help stabilise his sicken cells. Then one day in 2015, I was in the house, got up to give Mwansa his medication and I decided to read on the box. What I read that day again reduced me to tears.

I was worried for my child, and thought why on earth should my child be going through this? Mwansa was on X-jade and blood transfusion with this, he was at risk of having a lot of Iron in his blood which could bring other complications including liver damage. We were worried for him even though he was on close monitor.

Kennedy did not think of anymore kids because of what we went through, he felt like, we had enough. They could not find any donor in time and we looked at how our boy was suffering then I suggested we try for a baby and maybe the baby could be a donor.

Then I became pregnant in 2012. Kennedy was a bit uncomfortable not sure what will happen to the second child as every child has one chance in four to have sickle cell. If the second child gets it then we will be finished, no life at all. He felt like why on earth would I do this to him? He also questioned God as to why did he allow the pregnancy? As for me I left it all to God.

Blood Exchange

One day, Mwansa was not feeling well and we took him to Disney ward at Northampton General Hospital, your boy has a crisis and few hours later his condition worsened and he got transferred to

Birmingham children's hospital. The plan was to do blood exchange as he had a lot of sickle cells in his blood that was what made him so unwell so quickly. They had spoken about this procedure way back before he got this crisis because it was getting difficult to find a donor. Blood exchange is a procedure which involves slowly removing the person's blood and replacing it with fresh donor blood or plasma. The exchange transfusion tries to reduce the number of sickle cells in the blood as much as possible, but it does not make them disappear. This was why they kept his name on the transplant list even though it was taking long to find a donor. Blood exchange was just temporal measure.

Ambulance Encounter

Anyway, on the way in an ambulance I became unwell and the paramedics had 2 patients. I always moved with a BP machine. I asked the paramedics to check my BP and yes it was not right. I couldn’t sit up and there was only one patient bed which my baby was using, I leaned on one of the paramedics, I could see she was uncomfortable but she was really helping me. She held on to me all the way.

I could feel the panic in the Ambulance. I tried to reassure them that I would be fine. They made a call to the general hospital and they were redirected to take me first as Mwansa was a little stable than I was according to them. But I insisted to take Mwansa first to children's hospital. Of course, they didn't listen to me.

They took me to Birmingham General hospital and Mwansa to Birmingham children's hospital. I tried to call Kennedy and the phone was not going through. I called my friend and she managed to get hold of him. The hospital also called Kennedy to tell him that Mwansa was alone. Kennedy was on a train at the time and according to him he was so confused. What does he do, his pregnant wife is unwell in hospital and his small child is alone in another hospital? He went to the children's hospital and found the intensive support team with Mwansa and taking him to intensive care to be put in inducive coma for the second time in 3 years of his life. He got unwell so quickly while in hospital a very bad infection had affected his system. Few minutes later the boy was put on the breathing machine.

At the general hospital the doctors took long to attend to me, the nurses took the observations and put oxygen on me and put me on a bed. I was getting restless, thinking about how my son was doing alone and I nearly self-discharged. I asked for the forms and one of the cleaners came to me and said wait here let me go and see the doctor that could check on you. You don't want to create a bad record for yourself, I was not thinking about myself at the time all I wanted was to be with my baby. I waited for few minutes and the doctor came, they checked on me and discharged me. They called the Ambulance to take me to my son. I got there and found our boy in a state I didn't hope I would find him; I broke down.

Kennedy didn't tell me because he didn't want me to worry and my condition to worsen. Mwansa was on life support for 7 days. He got better and transferred to a general ward and back to Northampton. They didn't get to do blood exchange because of how things turned out to be.

Constant Worry

We were worried throughout my second pregnancy. We were worried of what it would be like if the second baby came out sickle cell positive on the other hand, we left it to God. The doctors suggested to see if the second baby would be a match by testing the placenta using an external agency that collects the placenta after birth.

His birth was also not straight forward because he was overdue by 10 days according to their calculation and I refused to be induced. According to my calculations he was not late. I told them I knew the due date and I would deliver normal. I asked them to give me until then as long as my baby was ok of which they agreed.

They said if I don't go in labour they will induce on that day. I agreed and they booked me in for 10am. About 3am I felt this pain, labour started on the day I said the baby would be born. We had arranged for child care, one of our friends from Milton Keynes came and picked up Mwansa and we headed to the hospital. We got to the hospital and the nurses thought I went to the arranged appointment but thankfully upon examination I was half dilated and Mwenya was born normal, praise be to God. The child screening took place, Sleepless nights continued and finally the results came in the letter confirming he was not positive. What a relief it was our God is faithful. We thanked God. The results for the placenta were not a match, what a shame! Mwansa continued to be on the register and on a lot of medication and regular blood transfusion increased, they monitored Iron levels because too much could bring more problems.

CHAPTER 5

Visit to Zambia

While waiting for the donor and Mwansa on regular transfusion. We visited Zambia for a month. The boys enjoyed and the last week before we came back, he developed mouth sores, Paul and kelvin took us to Chelstone clinic and we got some antibiotics from the nurse (We didn't get to the see doctor). When we got back to UK, we took him for check up and for his appointment which was booked before we left for Zambia. The consultant said the infection needed stronger antibiotics. They then tried to access the port but they couldn't.

They took X-ray and sent us home. We were walking home and just got to town (reached KFC in town) to be precise about 10 minutes from the Hospital, we received a call that we needed to go back as soon as possible. We thought something was not right and we were not wrong. It was a serious one that we didn't imagine. The ambulance was ready straight away to take the Mwansa to Birmingham children Hospital. Dr Koodiyedath took us in the cubical and said, the tube for the port had snapped and it had gone inside the heart through the left ventricle.

There was two options she said, they could use the key hole surgery or open heart surgery to take it out. Lord have Mercy it is too much for the poor boy. This was too much for Mwansa and for us, we were worried he might not make it but God was at the forefront. Kennedy went home to pack a few things to use and I went with the boy in the ambulance. The surgery was done and was successful shorter time than initially thought. Mwansa recovered well. And our journey with him continued.

CHAPTER 6

Marriage

We were newly married and still at the time when we were learning each other even though we dated for a long time. As you may know the early years in married can be challenging. This coupled with what we were going through with our son, our marriage lost signal or network. No or limited communication. I sometimes felt like I was trapped in a place with no air and light. I felt like there was no way out. I felt like maybe it was because we were alone with no family support and I felt the need to go back to Zambia. I questioned what I was doing in the UK. I felt like my life was on a stand still. Again, I would turn to God and say you know why you brought me this far.

We decided to go on separation. I didn't know whether to just take our sons to Zambia and stay there, but again Kennedy told me I wouldn't as he was the father and he will call the home office and tell them that I could not take my sons out of the country. I was worried of what could happen if I took Mwansa to Zambia. The medical system is totally different from the UK. One day I called our consultant and broke down on the phone. She asked me to go and see her in her office. I came out comforted. Sometimes you look at the doctors and think their jobs is just to make sure we are healthy but our consultant extended herself in helping with our personal issue and thanks to her we are here. She is one in a million. Every time we take our son for his appointments, she stops to check how we are doing, how we are coping with our sons. There's nothing with a price we can thank her with, that can show our gratitude but we only ask our God to bless her in abundance.

Church

I stopped going to church for over one year as I was just upset with everything that was happening. I didn't want people to talk to me about my issues, all I did was work and look after Mwansa and Mwenya.

My sisters would ask me to go to church and especially find a church that deals with healing and deliverance. My husband's family told him the same. One day we managed to sit and talk and we found a healing and deliverance Pastor Shadrack online. We called him and he prayed for us straight away and advised us to go to church on Sunday. I used to go to Jehovah's witnesses (though not at the time) but I decided to go and see the pastor. The pastor prayed for us and he said you are blocking a lot of blessings that God wants to bless you with by being separate and told us a lot of things that day but what I can say for now is we were back together and it was all God. We thank pastor Shadrack for his ministry.

Potential Donors

Few months later we received a phone call that 4 potential donors had been found from the United States but it was 9/10 match. We started the procedures with one of the donors. Consequently, Zika virus started and the potential donor who was young went to Brazil with his family and the area they visited was one of the zika virus affected areas and as such the procedure was suspended for another year and Mwansa was back on the donor register. Everything seemed to be on a stand still.

Bone Marrow Treatment

As they say everything happen for a reason, Kennedy was at work, he received a call from Birmingham children hospital that the potential donor had been found in south America who is 100% match. You need to bring your child to Birmingham on Wednesday to start the process, the person on the phone said. It was emotional such that Kennedy shed tears. Could it be that our differences and bitterness made the process to delay? (But again, delay is not denial).

Because he remembered Pastor Shadrack say if your heart is not at peace its very unlikely that God will move in your lives. You need to forgive and remain faithful then you will see what God can do in your lives and those of your loved ones. Then, he called and told me about the call, I was so thrilled and this reduced me to tears too. Kennedy spoke to his manager about the call and she was happy with the development and reassured him of the support she would afford.

According to Kennedy It made him reinforce his belief that, it's good to be good to people regardless. Kennedy did his best to support his manager and the manager was happy to help at the time of his need. He tries to be nice to people because so many people have been for us, just like we found ourselves here in the UK. It was because of people who are not even related to us. Thanks to The Late Dr Musanide, Hon Sichilima and Mr K Salati and Mr Nelson Oenga.

An appointment was booked to go for surgery to insert a central line. Mwansa was given a teddy bear to show him how the line will be fitted and how he will need to look after it, they also gave some bags to keep it in. He called the bear Agley. A central line is a type of catheter that is placed in a large vein that allows multiple IV fluids to be given and blood to be drawn. When compared to a typical IV line, a central line is larger, can stay in place longer, can deliver a greater volume of fluids and allows blood to be drawn easily.

This was in addition to the pot that he already had. We also had a call from Dr Lawson, that we were to take our son to oxford for testicle removal, they were to keep the testicles in case he didn't get to have children in future because of Chemotherapy and if it affected his fertility. During one of our appointments with the doctors we asked what would happen if Mwansa could not have children because of chemotherapy, we were told if he was older, it would have been easier as they keep their testicles and can give it back when they are older just as they keep girls eggs. Luckily for us that was the year they approved for under 10 to have their testicles kept. That evening the doctor called and Kennedy drove to oxford for the procedure. And as it is now Mwansa has part of his tescticles kept in Oxford Hospital and the Hospital will give it to him in future if need be. (God forbid all will be ok).

Moving to Hospital

Before we moved in, we met the psychologist. We discussed about ways to cope throughout the treatment. She asked whether we had any religious belief and we told her we were Christians and she was thrilled as she had never had problems with people that believes in God. That was our first and last we met as every time she called whether we wanted to see her we refused as we were ok. The nurse came and showed us where Mwansa was going to have his treatment from, what we needed to bring and how we needed to pack them as they take extra care to limit infections going to the ward, the nurse explained everything we needed to know during treatment. An appointment was made to move in.

Start of Treatment – First Chemotherapy

On 31/ 12/ 2016 we got admitted at Birmingham children's hospital ward 15 expected to be there for 3 months or more. This was the day Mwansa had started his 1 of 7 chemotherapy session.

The transplant starts with killing all your immune system and they use cancer medicine to do that. The experience was breath-taking. Any blood disorders such as Cancer, thalassemia, sickle cell were all treated in that ward. Mwansa was next to this cheerful boy who was there for cancer treatment and they started the treatment on the same day and they played together. On the second day, one of our bed neighbours informed us she lost her daughter and we thought of withdrawing from the treatment. We could not want to imagine coming out of the ward without Mwansa.

We told Mwansa, God is with you and you will be fine. He asked who is God we said the God who brought you in this world and the same God who saved your life. Ok Dad, he said.

On the second day in the evening, we were moved to the ward that has isolation rooms where he was not allowed to leave. To go through the doors only two carers were allowed and you had to wash your hands and leave the coats outside the rooms in the allocated drawers for each room. He was not allowed to be visited even by Mwenya his little brother, he was not allowed to meet his older brother for two weeks.

This was really hard for the boys as they are so close. The brother could only see him through the window. We were given a parent room to sleep in at

Ronald McDonald House and we took turns to look after our two boys. His and our clothes were washed in the isolation room. Showered twice a day using some antiseptic shower gel. Nothing was allowed in the room apart from the things we came in with.

Mwansa continued with chemotherapy and What was scary was that every time he had chemotherapy, he will be very weak and will spent the whole day sleeping. His appetite started to disappear. His mouth became sore and slowly struggled to eat and drink. His skin colour changed he became very dark, his hair started failing off, he would sleep on the pillow and the next thing is the whole hair on that side will be out and he would be asking why his hair came off. His dad cut the whole hair. His voice also changed, he spoke very softly.

He Continued to have chemotherapy till his immune level was 00 before they could transfuse with new born marrow cells. One thing he did even if he felt week is ask to play gospel songs and he always asked to call pastor Shadrack to pray. Thank God the pastor usually called to check up on him and pray. Mwansa would be in the bath and gospel songs would be playing. The nurses changed the beddings twice a day while in shower and they also listened to his music. The chemotherapy took its effect and he was tired and in bed all the time. But he always listened to gospel songs.

Bone Marrow Transfusion Day

Bone marrow (sometimes referred to as stem cell transplant) is just like blood transfusion. Mwansa finished his chemotherapy and the procedure was on as planned. On the 9th January 2017 everything was set for the transplant. Everyone was waiting for the bone marrow which was delayed to arrive. We were reassured that one of the transplant nurses will stay to make sure Mwansa receive it.

The born marrow arrived at Stansted airport a bit late and there was no specific time when it was getting to Birmingham. Anyway, thankfully one stem cell transplant nurse remained behind to carry out the procedure. Mid-afternoon the cells arrived, two nurses came to the room to do the procedure. The bone marrow was placed in a big 60 mls syringe and they pushed it very slowly into his tiny veins.

They explained that they harvested very good cell and he didn't need a big bag like one they put blood in and they didn't need to put it up to transfuse slowly as it was small. Within 10 minutes everything was over, it was just the matter of waiting for the cells to start its production. Every day, they checked his blood and for 52 days they took and tested his blood. Everything seemed to be going on well. The doctors initially thought he would have bad side effect as he was one of the patients that deteriorated very quickly but thankfully God is wonderful. He did not allow Mwansa to suffer too much.

One thing I feel bad even today is my husband missed the transplant. We planned that one will watch on the window while looking after Mwenya and the other would stay with Mwansa, but like I said because the born marrow arrived at Stansted airport a bit late and there was no specific time when it was getting to Birmingham, Kennedy decided to go and feed Mwenya and the bone mallow arrived in the middle of feeding and he couldn't stop. Thanks to technology I managed to record a video and Kennedy watched.

Another Surgery

The port cath stopped working for the third time since it was put in. The central line was also not working properly so they decided to insert another port. Our boy went to theatre to have an operation and all went well by God's grace. Mwansa was then allowed to move up and about in the isolation ward and he would ask to go for a walk, it was a big relief for him as he could now go out of his room which he had attempted to go out before he was allowed. Our boy would walk with fluids running and would be dancing to the music on the radio, he played doctor and the nurses laughed. They called him special patient as he responded to the treatment better than what they had initially anticipated.

My mother travelled from Zambia to help us look after the boys and it was a big relief. It was a big struggle for us, we had to work to be able to pay our bills, and we had to care for our two boys one that was in Birmingham Hospital and our jobs were in Northampton. Bless our Mwenya our second born, we moved him from here and there. He was constantly travelling between Birmingham and Northampton.

I had annual leave days and I asked to spread the days and only work 3 days a week. I would take him to Northampton so that I could work the 3 days, woke him up so early thanks to Petronella my friend, she would drop him off at nursery for me sometimes and I would get him after work. On the third day we would get the train back so that Kennedy can also go back to Northampton to work. The first 3 weeks it was ok as Kennedy's manager was so understanding. She gave him paid leave and so he did not travel back and forth.

Discharged

Living with a sickle cell child can be challenging, everything becomes difficult. Finances is one of it. We couldn't work properly as mostly we would be admitted in hospital. Life becomes somehow on hold. Mwansa got fed up of hospital and kept asking when we would go home. We then had an issue with the house, just before we went to Birmingham for treatment, we had a very big leek in the kitchen, the water came from the bathroom upstairs and this led to dampness and the moulds started. As a transplant patient he was not to go in a house with moulds or dust. Luckily the housing association found a house for us. Thanks to the consultant's input.

While sorting out the housing issue, the nurses started teaching us how to give medication, even though we were used to giving medication, they had to show us other things like how to check the acid levels as Mwansa initially had a gastric tube in his nose and there was a possibility he would be discharged with it. We finished signing the medication forms and instead of being in hospital for 3 months within 2 months Mwansa got discharged on a lot of medications.

On discharge Mwansa was not allowed take away foods and to go to public places for 3 months.

No school, no church, strict diet and we were to clean the house while he sat in another room and allowed the dust to settle before he could come out. We had to visit the hospital 3 times a week transport organised by the hospital.

Hospital Again

They continued to take bloods and unfortunately, 3 days later, the doctor called to say we needed to go back into the hospital. Devastating it was, only when we thought all looked ok and after being in there nearly 2 months. Reluctantly, Kennedy drove back this time to another ward. Mwansa developed a virus which needed intravenous medication. He stayed there and we took turns to stay with him. 3 weeks later we got discharged.

Taking It Slow

We stayed watchful and on tip toes, we kind of thought another call would come to go back to the hospital but that never happened. We continued to see the Doctors, it was reduced to twice a week, then once and then fortnightly and then monthly and then his medication kept on being reduced after every appointment. Then Mwansa' s hair started growing again like a baby. He was then allowed to eat take away but only MacDonald's and thankfully that's his best take away restaurant.

Because they had wiped all his immune system, Mwansa had to start his immunisations from one. All the baby immunisation was scheduled and he got them all. He was also allowed to travel within Europe. And in 2018 he went to Disney land Paris, facilitated by Just giving charity.

They now see him yearly and this will be for the rest of his life. He has passed his two years posttransplant and they have checked he is no longer a sickle cell patient. He has responded so well and never suffers like before. He can now visit anywhere in the world. Our God has done it for our boy and for us. It finally felt like we could now enjoy life. We could just plan of going somewhere without thinking about medications. Before this, we would go out even just to see a friend and our mind would be thinking about the time to give medications (He still takes Penicillin as prophylaxis because he has no spleen). We could not plan our holiday like any normal family. People buy tickets in advance to get them cheaper but we could not do that because of the uncertainty. What if we bought the tickets and Mwansa got unwell before we could travel? We had to get them few days before travelling.

We were also relieved as now we thought no more hospitals, we are one of the families that knows nearly every department in Northampton and Birmingham Hospital. Some people have never been in hospital with their children except when they went to have their children but for us Hospital was our second home. If we were asked to pay rent, we would not argue.

The nurses and doctors knew us and the moment you say you are Aaron's parent they knew and got ready for him. We would go there and sometimes more than five medical personnel would come to see him. This was also distressing for the doctors and it was not nice to see. Finally, we thought it was over.

CHAPTER 7

Another Baby

We asked Mwansa what his biggest gift could be and he said he would want another sibling especially twin sisters. We had a good laugh. As if it was not a lesson enough, we trusted God and decided to have a child. Few months after discharge I became pregnant. We hoped it would be a girl to fulfil our boy's wish but it turned out to be another boy. We then were worried about what it would be like if it was turned out to be a sickle cell baby. Throughout the pregnancy Mwansa kept saying it was girls even though we told him it was a boy, funny.

And our fears were true, baby Eirian Mayamiko was born with sickle cell and I clearly remember that phone call. We were driving to the hospital and the midwife called to say it was positive, he had sickle cell. We were listening to a gospel song and we both stayed quite for a while and after we just said why God? We were annoyed that we prayed for a baby girl and child with no sickle cell but none was given to us.

A day later we were calmer and said God has his own reasons and he has done it before and even Mayamiko will be fine. We apologised to God for questioning him. We are only humans and yes, we felt that way. Our God is a good God, he has forgiven us.

The Symptoms

Mayamiko started showing signs at the same age as was Mwansa. This time we had so much experience, we knew how to feel the spleen and we knew how to spot signs. Mayamiko started having the same complications that Mwansa had, one day he was crying of pain and when we checked him it was his fingers, they were swollen and we knew then it was a crisis.

We took him to the hospital and the doctors checked him and yes it was a crisis and they admitted us to observe him for a day. While at the hospital he developed a cough and he deteriorated very quickly. On the following morning they decided to scan his chest. They discovered he had water around his heart. This was even hard for the doctors as they were trying to work out how to make the water disappear, make sure he was well hydrated as he is a sickle cell patient, they did not want him to be dehydrated but they didn't want him to have too much water. They were in constant communication with Birmingham and they were planning to transfer him as Birmingham is a specialised Children's hospital and they have all the equipment if need be. It was a hard one for us also.

Mwansa got this unstoppable cough, he usually got it and normally will end up going to the hospital because the inhalers won't respond and the hospital used Nebuliser to control it. Mayamiko was in HDU (High Dependency Unit) at the time and Mwansa came in and was also admitted. They could not put him in another ward as Mwenya needed to be cared for at home and the doctors decided to bring Mwansa to HDU so that I could see them both. Because of the way he was coughing they decided to do some test and they found that he had an infection. They prescribed antibiotics and on the next day discharged him and gave us a day to take him back for review. The struggle with Mayamiko carried on and thanks to God he started responding to the treatment and we ended up not going to Birmingham.

Transplant

The doctors then decided to put him up for transplant as this was the same thing that used to happen to Mwansa. He would get really unwell and scare everyone. He was also put on hydroxycarbamide which has helped him. But the question has always been for how long can he depend on this strong medication? It is sometimes distressing for us. As for me I look at him and just wish I could do something that could take this sickle cell out of his system. I sometimes cry not knowing what next. Of course, Kennedy has no idea about this. I also have other children that I would not want them to see me crying. It is hard as a mother, but I just want the best for my children. I sometimes blame myself but again God knows. We were at some point told that a potential donor was found but the ratios were not very good. They wanted the same as what they got for Mwansa, 100%. We are hopeful and trust God is in control.

Luckily, at the time Eirian was born the Hospital had recruited a Haemoglobinopathies clinical specialist nurse, Claire Stockley. She has been a rock to us, she makes sure all is well with Eirian, she comes home to check up on him and take bloods. This is big relief as we do not take the other children with us to the hospital especially when one of us is working. She makes sure Eirian has regular appointments to see his consultant's Dr Koodiyedath and Dr Breene.

Sometimes we feel so lucky to have Dr Koodiyedath and Dr Breene. They are always there for us. There are days when Eirian will be unwell and they will be holding their clinic, they will make sure they take a break to come and asses our boy. They cannot let him go home before they see him. This was the case with Mwansa. We are just so grateful. Sometimes we feel sorry for them because you could see they are tired and they need a rest but they are there to make sure our boy was well. If we had a biggest gift in the world to give it would go to them. But we can only ask our God to bless them.

The nurses also have been so helpful to us, especially the nurses from Disney ward. They now know us and they did not judge us when they heard we had another child with sickle cell. You could see they were happy that we had a child and they are always happy to help.

With Mwansa, one of the male nurses from Disney ward told us never to take Mwansa to the GP but to take him straight to Disney as Mwansa sometime got unwell at the time we spent at the GP and the GP will end up sending us to the hospital and this is what we do for Eirian, we take him straight to the hospital and the nurses are always happy to help. We cannot thank them enough.

Fourth Baby

Few months after the birth Mayamiko I became pregnant, our God has a plan. Again, this turned out to be a boy. So, we now have four boys. As usual they tested to check whether he had sickle cell and thank God for this he is free from sickle cell and has no trace. They took blood samples to test whether he was a match. The results came back and unfortunately, he is also not a match. We continue to be hopeful a match will be found. We named him Gavi (God is our strength) Chimwemwe (praise, thank God) as God is our only strength. He has always been there even at our weakest time.

You're Strong

Some people say I am such a strong person as I have dealt with this situation so well. They don't know I have been at my lowest and have cried more than anyone should. Not even my husband realised this. The only thing that keeps me going is the belief I have in God and that he sees our suffering. He will for sure one day put a stop to our suffering. I believe God has given us boys for a big reason which one day he will show. All my siblings have at least girls and boys but I got all boys. God never does things without a purpose and his purpose will one day be seen. I am the only one with children with sickle cell even in my extended family, I believe God has a reason for this as well.

I had a kind of a glimpse to it. In January 2020, doctors had what they called East Midlands Sickle cell and Thalassemia Network |(EMSTN) education day and they invited us to go and give an experience of what it is like living with children with sickle cell. We were the only parents there and all were doctors.

We were chosen because of what we have been through and we were chosen to help other doctors understand the real struggle that is there and so they could make the needed improvements.

We do appreciate all the efforts the doctors make, now no sickle cell child will have to wait to be seen by the doctors. They have put a time frame between arrival and the time they should be seen.

This will reduce on the children's and parents' distress. I remember when our child stopped breathing and when we finally spoke to people about it, they normally advised to sue the hospital so that they should change the way they operate but we said there was another way to this and not to drag people to courts.

The doctors did their best that night to keep our boy alive and we thank God for them for that but we did not want to put anyone in distress. Thank God another way came, we managed to speak to doctors and for sure they implemented some of the things we mentioned.

Other Challenges

Financial struggle is another thing, as we could not work properly. We were always on strict budgets as we did not know what the next day will be like. I might be at work and the nursery would call because Mwansa was not well and that might take a week with no work and no income. Sleepless nights, when Mwansa and Mayamiko were unwell, even when they are ok, we are constantly worried what the next day will be like. We could not plan a normal holiday like every normal family do. We have to stay put because even if Mwansa is ok we have Eirian to think about. Even after Mwansa's treatment we have not felt like we can take Eirian anywhere as we are still worried what it could be like.

The struggle with child care is another, one had to stay at the hospital and the other with the other children meaning we couldn't spend time as a family and this brought a strain on our relationship. This has now improved because we found friends that have turned to be our family. My friend Chitalu and the mother Prosperlyn who we now also call mum have been there for us. My other friend Petronella.

They have supported us like they are our blood relatives. They are always rushing when we call for help, child care has also been easy as the boys know them as family and are happy to spend a night at their house. Elizabeth our neighbour has also been helpful, she helps with school runs when one of the boys is in hospital or has an appointment with the doctors.

Mwansa started reception and we were worried as to how he would cope. On most days, the teachers would report that he was very tired, his energy levels were normally low because his hb (Haemoglobin) was usually below 90. Cold weather would make the skin swollen like bee hives, he would go to play outside like any other child and his face would swell. We advised the teachers not to take him out when it was cold and this was difficult with the school as they had to have a teacher remain in class with him, he moved to year one and the report of concentration came in. Because he felt tired most of the times, it was difficult for him to concentrate throughout his lessons but thank God this is not an issue now after his treatment. We worry for Eirian now and hope it will not be like that.

Finding a donor was and has been a challenge. I say so because it took a long time to find a perfect donor for Mwansa and it has taken long to find a donor for Eirian. We have very few people especially from ethnic group that have registered to be donors. We were tested as a family and non has turned out to be a match. We are begging people to please register with Anthony Nolan and also DMDK Registry to be able to help someone not just sickle cells sufferers but also other blood disorders sufferers. The procedure to donate your cells does not hurt and it will help save lives.

I have heard from a number of people that were asked to have sickle cell screening in their pregnancy and accepted but after the positive result they were faced with a choice of either to keep or to terminate. And they all went for the later, if we had people registering for stem cell donation maybe they would not have terminated their babies. They would have that hope that their children will get the treatment. We fully understand it can be very expensive for the NHS to do the procedure. But again, a child is a gift from God and we are expected to appreciate God for what we are given. It is not a choice to have a child with an illness. There are people all over the world that dream of getting pregnant and have a child. But others get pregnant so easily and end up terminating for the unknown fear.

If you are faced with that choice today, I would encourage you to leave it to God. Keep the baby and leave it to God to handle it. He has given you that child and he will see you through. The bible tells us God will not allow you to be tempted beyond what you can bear but he will always provide a way out for you. Stay strong and trust God. If I had a way to stop this screening, I would definitely stop it because I have spoken to people that went through it and ended up terminating and later regrated and that started eating them up, also others that went through it got a positive result and decided to terminate a baby that they got to see and until today they regret. Yes, this is to give a chance to parents that feel they can not cope but the after effect is not good.

For young people looking for love, I would advise you to get checked and always ask the other person whether they know their sickle cell status because it is not easy to look after a sick child. You really want to enjoy your life with kids and not to be visiting hospitals.

We have not had a donor for our Eirian but we believe and trust God will deal with it, the God that did it for Mwansa will do it for Eirian. Our boys get unwell quite often but we jump on increased antibiotic quickly and this has been because of the experience with Mwansa. We usually contact his consultant when this happens. Honestly, living with a sick child is not easy. Even just a simple cough will worry you.

Now Covid 19 has come in and the fear has worsened. Sometimes you feel guilty for not allowing friends to come in the house but again you are trying to protect your children. I had someone say to me that I have taken this Covid 19 too seriously, that I needed to loosen up a bit. They clearly did not understand what we go through and I can only ignore and forgive them as they have no idea what it is like to live with an illness.

Our God has been our strength through it all. He moved us from Africa because he was preparing us for this. The story would have been so much different if we were in Africa. We feel for parents in Africa because of the health service there. The doctors and nurses have also played a very bigger role in our lives and we ask our creator to bless them abundantly. If you are going through the same, know that God will always be there and you will come out of your situation. Work with the doctors as God works through people. May God be your strength in all you are passing through. Peace be with you. Scripture 1 Corinthians 10:13.

THE END

Aaron is a young boy, who had severe sickle cell complications. He was only about 6 months when he first experienced what is called sickle cell crisis. It was very severe that he stopped breathing and had to be resuscitated. He suffered many more crisis throughout his first years of life up until he got treated using stem cells.

Eirian is Aaron's brother who also has sickle cell and also experienced his first crisis at the same age as Aaron did, at only about 6 months. He started having quite a lot of complications and thanks to the advancement in medicine, the doctors decided to start him early on Hydroxycarbamide which has helped stabilise his sickle a little. Although the question for us has always been for how long can he take this medication?

The book details the struggles that the children and us as parent have gone through.

We hope you enjoy reading.

www.ingramcontent.com/pod-product-compliance
Lightning Source LLC
LaVergne TN
LVHW021301160826
845679LV00001B/161

9798356840548